NOURISHING HOPE

A Personalized Diet Guide for Chron's Disease Patients to Restore Health and Wellbeing

JAMES HALEN

Contents

Introduction

Crohn's disease is a type of inflammatory bowel disease (IBD). As many as 780,000 Americans have the condition, according to the Crohn's & Colitis Foundation of America (CCFA).

More research about Crohn's disease is necessary. Researchers aren't sure how it begins, who is most likely to develop it, or how to best manage it. Despite major treatment advances in the last 3 decades, no cure is available yet.

Crohn's disease most commonly occurs in the small intestine and the colon. It can affect any part of your gastrointestinal (GI) tract, from the mouth to the anus. It can involve some parts of the GI tract and skip other parts.

The range of severity for Crohn's is mild to debilitating. Symptoms vary and can change over time. In severe cases, the disease can lead to life threatening flares and complications.

Here's everything you need to know about Crohn's disease.

Crohn's symptoms

The symptoms of Crohn's disease often develop gradually. Certain symptoms may also become worse over time. Although it's possible, it's rare for symptoms to develop suddenly and dramatically. The earliest symptoms of Crohn's disease can include:

• diarrhea

• abdominal cramps

• blood in your stool

• fever

• fatigue

• loss of appetite

• weight loss

• feeling as if your bowels aren't empty after a bowel movement

• feeling a frequent need for bowel movements

It's sometimes possible to mistake these symptoms for those of another condition, such as food poisoning, an upset stomach, or an allergy. You should see your doctor if any of these symptoms persist.

The symptoms may become more severe as the disease progresses. More troublesome symptoms may include:

9

• a perianal fistula, which causes pain and drainage near your anus

• ulcers that may occur anywhere from the mouth to the anus

• inflammation of the joints and skin

• shortness of breath or decreased ability to exercise due to anemia

Early detection and diagnosis can help you avoid severe complications and allow you to begin treatment early.

What causes Crohn's disease?

It isn't clear what causes Crohn's disease. However, the following factors may influence your chances of developing it:

• your immune system

• your genes

• your environment

Up to 20 percent of people with Crohn's disease also have a parent, child, or sibling with the disease, according to the CCFA.

According to a 2012 study, certain factors can affect the severity of your symptoms. These include:

• whether you smoke

• your age

• whether or not the rectum is involved

• length of time you've had the disease

People with Crohn's are also more likely to develop intestinal infections from bacteria, viruses, parasites, and fungi. This can affect the severity of symptoms and create complications.

Crohn's disease and its treatments can also affect the immune system, making these types of infections worse.

Yeast infections are common in Crohn's and can affect both the lungs and the intestinal tract. It's important that these infections are diagnosed and properly treated with antifungal medications to prevent further complications.

Crohn's diagnosis

No single test result is enough for your doctor to diagnose Crohn's disease. They will begin by eliminating other possible causes of your symptoms.

Your doctor may use several types of tests to make a diagnosis:

• Blood tests can help your doctor look for certain indicators of potential problems, such as anemia and inflammation.

• A stool test can help your doctor detect blood in your GI tract.

• Your doctor may request an endoscopy to get a better image of the inside of your upper gastrointestinal tract.

• Your doctor may request a colonoscopy to examine the large bowel.

• Imaging tests like CT scans and MRI scans give your doctor more detail than an average X-ray. Both tests allow your doctor to see specific areas of your tissues and organs.

• Your doctor will likely have a tissue sample, or biopsy, taken during an endoscopy or colonoscopy for a closer look at your intestinal tract tissue.

Once your doctor has completed reviewing all the necessary tests and ruled out other possible reasons for your symptoms, they may conclude that you have Crohn's disease.

Your doctor may go on to request these tests several more times to look for affected tissue and determine how the disease is progressing.

The Healthline FindCare tool can provide options in your area if you need help finding a primary care doctor or a gastroenterologist.

Treatment for Crohn's disease

A cure for Crohn's disease isn't available yet, but the disease can be managed. Variety of treatment options exist that can lessen the severity and frequency of your symptoms.

Medications

Several types of medications are available to treat Crohn's. Antidiarrheal and anti-inflammatory drugs are commonly used. More advanced options include biologics, which use the body's immune system to treat the disease.

The medications, or combination of medications, you need depend on your symptoms, your disease history, the severity of your condition, and how you respond to treatment.

Anti-inflammatory drugs

The two main types of anti-inflammatory drugs doctors use to treat Crohn's are oral 5-aminosalicylates and corticosteroids. Anti-inflammatory drugs are often the first drugs you take for Crohn's disease treatment.

You typically take these drugs when you have mild symptoms with infrequent disease flares.

Corticosteroids are used for more severe symptoms but should only be taken for a short time.

Immunomodulators

An overactive immune system causes the inflammation that leads to the symptoms of Crohn's disease. Drugs that affect the immune system, called immunomodulators, may reduce the inflammatory response and limit your immune system's reaction.

Antibiotics

Some doctors believe antibiotics may help reduce some of the symptoms of Crohn's and some of the possible triggers for it.

For example, antibiotics can reduce drainage and heal fistulas, which are abnormal connections between tissues that Crohn's can cause.

Biologic therapies

If you have severe Crohn's, your doctor may try one of a number of biologic therapies to treat the inflammation and complications that can occur from the disease. Biologic drugs can block specific proteins that may trigger inflammation.

Surgery

If less invasive treatments and lifestyle changes don't improve your symptoms, surgery may be necessary. Ultimately, about 75 percent of people with Crohn's disease will require surgery at some point in their lives, according to the CCFA.

Some types of surgery for Crohn's include removing damaged portions of your digestive tract and reconnecting the healthy sections. Other procedures repair damaged tissue, manage scar tissue, or treat deep infections.

Diet

Food doesn't cause Crohn's disease, but it can trigger flares.

After a Crohn's diagnosis, your doctor will likely suggest making an appointment with a registered dietitian (RD). An RD will help you understand how food may affect your symptoms and how your diet may help you.

In the beginning, they may ask you to keep a food diary. This food diary will detail what you ate and how it made you feel.

Using this information, the RD will help you create an eating plan. These dietary changes should help you absorb more nutrients from the food you eat while also limiting any negative side effects food may be causing.

Crohn's disease diet

A diet plan that works for one person with Crohn's disease may not work for another. This is because the disease can involve different areas of the GI tract in different people.

It's important to find out what works best for you. This can be done by keeping track of your symptoms as you add or remove certain foods from your diet. Lifestyle and diet changes may help you reduce the recurrence of symptoms and lessen their severity.

Adjust fiber intake

Some people need a high fiber, high protein diet. For others, the presence of extra food residue from high fiber foods such as fruits and vegetables may aggravate the GI tract. If this is the case, you may need to switch to a low residue diet.

On this particular diet has been mixed, so speak with your doctor about your personal needs.

Limit fat intake

Crohn's disease may interfere with your body's ability to break down and absorb fat. This excess fat will pass from your small intestine to your colon, which can cause diarrhea.

However, a 2017 study on mice suggested that a diet higher in plant-based fats had the potential to change the gut microbiome in positive ways for Crohn's disease. More research is needed and your doctor or an RD can help guide you in your fat intake.

Limit dairy intake

Previously, you may not have experienced lactose intolerance, but your body can develop difficulty digesting some dairy products when you have Crohn's disease. Consuming dairy can lead to an upset stomach, abdominal cramps, and diarrhea for some people.

Drink enough water

Crohn's disease may affect your body's ability to absorb water from your digestive tract. This can lead to dehydration. The risk of dehydration is especially high if you're having diarrhea or bleeding.

Consider alternative sources of vitamins and minerals

Crohn's disease can affect your intestines' ability to properly absorb other nutrients from your food. Eating nutrient-dense foods may not be enough. Talk with your doctor about taking multivitamins to find out if this is right for you.

Work with your doctor to figure out what best suits your needs. They may refer you to an RD or nutritionist. Together, you can identify your dietary plan and create guidelines for a balanced diet.

Natural treatments for Crohn's

Some people use complementary and alternative medicine (CAM) to help manage symptoms of various conditions and diseases, including Crohn's disease.

The Food and Drug Administration hasn't approved these for treatment, but some people use them in addition to mainstream medications.

Don't add any new treatments to your current treatment plan without consulting your doctor.

Some CAM treatments for Crohn's disease include:

• Probiotics. These are live bacteria that can help you replace and rebuild the good bacteria in your intestinal tract. Probiotics may also help prevent microorganisms from upsetting your gut's natural balance and causing a Crohn's flare. Scientific data about effectiveness is limited.

• Prebiotics. These are potentially beneficial materials found in plants, such as asparagus, bananas, artichokes, and leeks, that help feed the good bacteria in your gut and increase their numbers.

• Fish oil. Fish oil is rich in omega-3s. According to a 2017 study, research is ongoing regarding its possible treatment of Crohn's disease. Oily fish like salmon and mackerel are rich in omega-3s. You can find fish oil supplements online.

• Supplements. Many people believe certain herbs, vitamins, and minerals ease the symptoms of a variety of diseases, including inflammation associated with Crohn's disease. Research is ongoing as to which supplements may be beneficial.

• Aloe vera. Some believe that the aloe vera plant has anti-inflammatory properties. Because inflammation is one of the key components of Crohn's disease, people may use it as a natural anti-inflammatory. However, there is no current research that suggests aloe vera helps with Crohn's.

• Acupuncture. This is the practice of strategically sticking needles in the skin to stimulate various points on the body. A 2014 study found that acupuncture, combined with moxibustion — a type of traditional Chinese medicine that involves burning dried medicinal herbs on or near your skin — improves symptoms of Crohn's disease. More research is needed.

Tell your doctor if you use any CAM treatments or over-the-counter medications. Some of these substances can affect the efficiency of medications or other treatments. In some cases, an interaction or side effect could be dangerous, or even life threatening.

Crohn's surgery

Surgery for Crohn's disease is considered a last-resort treatment, but three-quarters of people with Crohn's will ultimately need some type of surgery to relieve symptoms or complications.

Once medications are no longer working or side effects have become too severe to treat, your doctor may consider one of the following surgeries.

• Stricture plasty widens and shortens the intestines in an attempt to reduce the effects of scarring or damage to the tissue.

• During a bowel resection, portions of damaged intestine are removed. Healthy intestine is stitched together to reform the intestines.

• An ostomy creates a hole through which your body can eliminate waste. These are usually performed when a portion of the small or large bowel is removed. They can be permanent or temporary when your doctor wants to give your intestines time to heal.

• A colectomy removes sections of the colon that are diseased or damaged.

• A proctocolectomy is surgery to remove the colon and rectum. If you have this surgery, you will also need a colostomy (a hole in the large intestine for emptying waste).

Crohn's disease surgery is helpful for relieving symptoms, but it's not without risk. Talk with your doctor about any concerns you may have with surgery.

What are the variations of Crohn's disease?

There are six variations of Crohn's disease, all based on location in the digestive system. They are:

• Gastroduodenal Crohn's disease. This uncommon condition mainly affects your stomach and the duodenum, which is the first part of your small intestine.

• Jejunoileitis. This type occurs in the second portion of your intestine, called the jejunum. Like gastroduodenal Crohn's, this variation is less common.

• Ileitis. Ileitis involves inflammation in the last part of the small intestine, or ileum.

• Ileocolitis. This affects the ileum and the colon and is the most common variation of Crohn's.

• Crohn's colitis. This affects the colon only. Both ulcerative colitis and Crohn's colitis impact the colon only, but Crohn's colitis can affect deeper layers of the intestinal lining.

• Perianal disease. This often involves fistulas, or abnormal connections between tissues, deep tissue infections, as well as sores and ulcers on the outer skin around the anus.

Crohn's disease and ulcerative colitis

Crohn's disease and ulcerative colitis (UC) are two types of IBD. They have many of the same characteristics. You may even mistake them for one another.

They have the following characteristics in common:

• The first signs and symptoms of both Crohn's disease and UC are very similar. These can include diarrhea, abdominal pain and cramping, rectal bleeding, weight loss, and fatigue.

• Both UC and Crohn's disease occur more commonly in people ages 15 to 35 and people with a family history of either type of IBD.

• In general, IBD tends to affect all sexes equally, but this can vary depending on age.

• Despite decades of research, scientists still don't know what causes either disease. In both cases, an overactive immune system is a likely culprit, but other factors likely play a role.

Here's how they differ:

• UC only affects the colon. Crohn's disease can affect any part of your GI tract, from the mouth to the anus.

• UC only affects the outermost layer of tissue lining your colon called the mucosa. Crohn's disease can affect all the layers of your intestinal tissue from superficial to deep.

UC is just one type of colon inflammation. Several other types of colitis exist. Not all forms of colitis cause the same type of intestinal inflammation and damage as UC.

Crohn's disease statistics

The CCFA and the Centers for Disease Control and Prevention (CDC) report the following statistics:

• Around 3 million Americans have some form of IBD. This total includes over 780,000 Americans who have Crohn's disease.

• People who actively smoke are twice as likely to receive a diagnosis of Crohn's disease.

• If the condition is treated — medically or surgically — 50 percent of people with Crohn's disease will go into remission or experience only mild symptoms within 5 years of their diagnosis.

• About 11 percent of people who have Crohn's will experience a chronically active disease.

The CCFA also reports:

• In 2004, 1.1 million doctors' office visits were for the treatment and care of Crohn's disease.

• In 2010, Crohn's disease accounted for 187,000 hospitalizations.

• The average person with Crohn's disease will spend between $8,265 and $18,963 annually to treat or manage their disease, per 2003–04 U.S. insurance claims data.

According to 2016 data:

• Crohn's disease occurs about as frequently in men as in women.

• Two out of three individuals with Crohn's disease will receive a diagnosis before the age of 40.

Meeting others within the Crohn's community can be extremely helpful. IBD Healthline is a free app that connects you with others who understand what you're going through via one-on-one messaging, live group discussions, and expert-approved information on managing IBD.

Crohn's disease and disability

Crohn's disease can disrupt your work and personal life. It can also cause financial stress. If you don't have health insurance (and sometimes even if you do), your out-of-pocket expenses can total several thousand dollars per year.

If the disease becomes severe enough that it's affecting your daily life in a significant way, consider filing for disability.

If you can prove that your condition prevents you from working or has prevented you from working for the last year, you may be eligible to receive disability income. Social Security Disability Insurance or Social Security Income can provide this type of assistance.

Unfortunately, applying for disability can be a long and tedious process. It requires lots of appointments with your doctors. You may have to pay for multiple doctors' visits if you don't have insurance. You'll need to take time off of work if you're currently employed.

Be aware that you may face a lot of ups and downs as you work through the process. You might even be denied and have to begin the whole process again. If you feel it's the right choice for you, you can begin your

Social Security application process by doing one of the following:

• Apply online.

• Call the Social Security Administration's toll-free hotline.

• Find and visit your nearest Social Security office.

Crohn's disease in children

Most people with Crohn's disease receive a diagnosis in their 20s and 30s, but IBD can develop in children, too. Approximately 1 in 4 people with an IBD show symptoms before age 20, according to a 2016 review.

Crohn's disease that only involves the colon is common in children and adolescents. That means distinguishing between Crohn's and UC is difficult until the child begins showing other symptoms.

Proper treatment for Crohn's disease in children is important because untreated Crohn's can lead to growth delays and weakened bones. It may also cause significant emotional distress at this stage in life. Treatments include:

- antibiotics

- aminosalicylates

- biologics

- immunomodulators

- steroids

- nutrition plans

Crohn's medications can have some significant side effects on children. It's vital you work closely with your child's doctor to find the right options.

Outlook

Research is still ongoing to find more effective treatments and potentially an eventual cure for Crohn's disease. But symptoms can be successfully managed and remission is possible.

Your doctor can help guide you in finding the right medications, alternative treatments, and lifestyle measures that can help.

If you're having gastrointestinal symptoms, speak with your doctor to determine the cause and potential solutions.

Recipe

BUCKWHEAT CREPES

Ingredients:

1 cup of buckwheat

1⁄2 cup flour rice

1⁄2 teaspoon salt

11⁄2 cups filtered water

Coconut spray oil

(Crepe pan needed for this recipe.)

Directions

Mix all the ingredients in a medium bowl by hand. Cover the bowl and let it rest overnight in the fridge. The next day, generously spray a crepe pan with coconut spray oil and place on medium heat. Spoon enough crepe mix into the pan to cover the entire surface. Cook the crepe for about one minute, until it appears to almost cook all the way through. Flip it over for 15 seconds, then remove. Fill your crepes with your favorite fillings, or eat plain.

Tip: These crepes freeze well; just place parchment paper between each one before placing it in a freezer bag. Remove one at a time and warm in the microwave for 30 seconds.

Another shout out to my mama—she created this recipe for me a couple months ago. It is a delicious, gluten free alternative to crepes. Did you know that buckwheat is derived from the seeds of a flowering plant?

BEST TASTING POWER PROTEIN BARS

Ingredients:

11/2 cups rice crisp cereal

1/4 cup sunflower seeds, half ground

1/4 cup pumpkin seeds, half ground

2 tablespoons sesame seeds

2 tablespoons hemp seeds

8 scoops or servings protein powder (whey, soy, rice or other protein powder alternative)

1/2 teaspoon sea salt

11/2 cups almond butter 11/2 cups brown rice syrup 1 teaspoon vanilla extract

Prepare a greased 9 × 9 or 9 × 13 baking pan or simply line the pan with 2 layers of wax paper. In a separate bowl, mix all dry ingredients together. Warm the almond butter and brown rice syrup in a saucepan over medium heat until it becomes soft and fluid. Add vanilla extract, pour over dry ingredients, and begin working mixture with your hands into a large clump.

Thoroughly mix the mixture to evenly coat the entire dry mix. Press tightly into greased pan or wax paper lined pan and chill in refrigerator until hard.

Once hard, cut into squares and store in an airtight container. These can very easily be stored in the freezer and taken out a few hours before enjoying.

These bars make excellent alternatives for breakfast and snacks on the go. Be careful—these are so good, they're almost addictive! Also, this recipe tends to vary depending on the liquid content of the almond butter and the quality and texture of the protein powder, so you may need to alter the amount of liquid, depending on how well the mixture stays together during the hand mixing process.

GLUTEN-FREE BANANA GRANOLA PANCAKES

Ingredients:

11/2 cups gluten-free pancake or baking mix 2 bananas, ripe

1 teaspoon vanilla extract

3/4 cup hemp milk

1/2 teaspoon baking soda

1/2 teaspoon cinnamon

1 cup granola

Directions

Heat lightly oiled skillet to medium heat. Add bananas, vanilla, and milk to blender and blend until smooth. Add baking soda, cinnamon, and half of the baking mix and blend until smooth. Add the second half of the baking mix and blend until smooth. Remove blender, add granola to the

mixture and stir in with a mixing spoon. Do not blend. Pour batter into 3-inch diameter circles in the pan. When the pancakes start to bubble, flip them carefully and cook on the other side until lightly browned on both sides.

BLUEBERRY SYRUP

Ingredients:

2 cups organic blueberries Stevia, to taste

Directions

Take two cups of blended blueberries and strain to remove seeds. Cook on low heat and stir frequently to form a light syrup. Cool slightly and sweeten with pure Stevia to taste. Serve over pancakes or light desserts.

EASY PANCAKES WITH GROUND PUMPKIN AND SUNFLOWER SEEDS

Ingredients:

3 tablespoons ground pumpkin seeds

3 tablespoons ground sunflower seeds

3 organic eggs

1/4 cup non-gluten flour

1/4 cup hemp milk, or other alternative milk 1/4 cup uncooked millet (optional)

1/4 cup blueberries (optional)

2 teaspoons baking soda

Heat lightly oiled skillet to medium heat. Combine all ingredients except blueberries and millet into a medium-sized bowl and mix well until clumps have dissolved. Add blueberries and/or millet if you are going to use these ingredients. Pour batter into 3-inch diameter circles in the pan. When pancakes start to bubble, flip them carefully and cook on the other side until lightly browned on both sides.

OATMEAL FOR ONE

Ingredients:

1/3 cup gluten-free rolled oats

1/3 cup light coconut milk from a can (alternative: almond milk, rice milk, water)

1/3 cup water

1/4 teaspoon cinnamon powder

1/2 teaspoon vanilla extract

1/2 organic banana, cut into thin slices Pinch of salt

Place all the ingredients in a medium size pot and place on medium-low heat. Simmer for 7 to 10 minutes, stirring every minute. Once the oats have absorbed most of the liquids and gained a creamy consistency, it will be done. If you like it very creamy, add more coconut milk. Serve and eat immediately.

Tip: Use honey as an optional topping to make this dish a bit sweeter, and top with your favorite crushed nuts.

I love eating oatmeal for breakfast. You can also cook this recipe in the microwave by placing all the ingredients in a bowl and heating it for 2 minutes. Cook longer if not at desired consistency. This is one of my go-to breakfasts that I take to work.

SMOOTHIE FOR ONE

Ingredients:

1/3 cup frozen organic blueberries

4–5 frozen organic strawberries

1 ripe organic banana

2 cubes of frozen dandelion, cilantro, and kale

1 hefty tablespoon of flaxseed powder

1 cup light coconut milk (water, almond milk, or plain rice milk) 1/2 cup filtered water

Directions

Place all the ingredients in the blender and blend. I like to blend mine to a liquid consistency to insure that everything is broken down, allowing less work for my digestive system. If you like it thicker, go ahead and add 3/4 of the liquids and add more from there until you get desired consistency.

I start every day with a smoothie. Any blender will do to make this smoothie. Once you get the hang of making the smoothie, you can begin to alter it to suite your taste buds and needs. If any of the fruits or vegetables I suggested bother you, don't add it or substitute something you find belly friendly for it. I juice 1 bunch of organic kale, 2 bunches of organic dandelion, and 2 bunches of organic cilantro at the beginning of each week and freeze them in ice cube trays. I use them throughout the week for my smoothies. All three have amazing anti- inflammatory properties.

TIP: DO YOU SOAK YOUR ALMONDS AND WALNUTS?

This is something I learned this past year: if you eat walnuts or almonds, you should be soaking them first. The top ten reasons why you should soak your nuts, along with your grains and seeds:

1. To remove or reduce phytic acid.

2. To remove or reduce tannins.

3. To neutralize the enzyme inhibitors.

4. To encourage the production of beneficial enzymes.

41

5. To increase the amounts of vitamins, especially B vitamins.

6. To break down gluten and make digestion easier.

7. To make the proteins more readily available for absorption.

8. To prevent mineral deficiencies and bone loss.

9. To help neutralize toxins in the colon and keep the colon clean.

10. To prevent many health diseases and conditions.

So what do you have to do? If you plan on eating almonds or walnuts, soak them in a bowl of filtered water, ensuring the water covers a couple inches above the nuts, as the nuts will expand as they absorb the water. Rinse them out well the next day (7 to 24 hours later) and enjoy. Make sure to peel the skin before you eat it. That skin can be tough on us to digest, even when soaked.

SPINACH, MUSHROOM, AND GOAT CHEESE EGG MUFFINS

Contributed by Sarah Choueiry

Ingredients:

1/2 (6-ounce) bag of organic spinach

1 cup organic button mushrooms, chopped

10 organic eggs

1/3 cup goat cheese, crumbled (optional)

1/2 teaspoon salt (add 1/2 teaspoon more if you are not adding the goat cheese)

1/2 teaspoon pepper

Directions

Preheat the oven to 375°F. Spray a frying pan with a nonstick spray and place on medium heat. Add the spinach and cook until softened. Once done, place the pan to the side. Crack 10 eggs into a large bowl, add salt and pepper, and whisk.

Line a muffin tin with 12 muffin cups. Spray each muffin cup with nonstick spray. Evenly distribute the spinach and mushrooms on the bottom of each muffin cup and pour in the egg liquid. Top with goat cheese. Once done, place the tin in the oven for approximately 25 minutes, until lightly browned on top.

Tip: For storing, wait 30 minutes, until they are cooled, before sticking them into the fridge. I store them in Tupperware. You can pop them in the microwave for 30 seconds and enjoy it the next day for your breakfast on the go!

I first came up with this recipe when hosting a brunch for my family. I wanted an easy dish to serve that did not take too much time to prepare, but was something I could eat. The nice thing about this recipe is that it is very flexible, so feel free to remove any suggested items and add your own.

BAKED EGGS IN AVOCADO

Ingredients:

1 large, ripe avocado

2 organic eggs

Salt and pepper, to taste

Directions

Preheat the oven to 425°F. Cut the avocado in half and remove the pit. You may have to scoop out a little of the avocado to ensure you have plenty of room for the egg. Crack one of the eggs directly into the hole in the avocado then repeat with the other avocado half. Place each half into small ramekins or other similar ovenware to ensure that the egg won't spill out. Top with salt and pepper to taste and bake for 15 minutes. Check to make sure the egg is cooked to your liking. Cook more if needed.

Randi's tip: This recipe leaves a lot of room to be creative; tons of other ingredients would be absolutely delicious atop this avocado slash egg haven. Some ideas are bacon, hot sauce, and scallions. Also, I spoon the avocado egg mix onto whole-wheat toast, but if your belly prefers to be gluten-free, try gluten-free bread or even a gluten-free cracker!

This recipe was created by Randi Howry, a chef and ulcerative colitis thriver. Randi has contributed amazing recipes to The Crohn's Journey Foundation that are gluten-free, dairy-free, and sugar-free. The recipes included in this book are some of my favorites.

SUNNY MORNING BURRITO

Serves 1

Ingredients:

1/4 cup chopped vegetables

1 egg

1 (6-inch) tortilla

1 tablespoon salsa (optional)

1/2 tablespoon light sour cream (optional)

In a small nonstick skillet, lightly sauté the chopped vegetables. Add the egg; stir to scramble. Cook until dry. Heat tortilla between wet paper towels for 30 seconds in the microwave. Tortillas can also be heated in the oven by wrapping in aluminum foil and baking at 350°F for 5 minutes. Tortillas roll more easily when warm. Fill tortilla with the egg and vegetable mixture. Serve with salsa or low-fat sour cream, if desired.

Leftover vegetables work well in this recipe. Use several kinds of vegetables (it is okay if you use more than the 1/4 cup). To reduce cholesterol, replace the egg with an egg substitute or two egg whites.

ZUCCHINI BUCKWHEAT BANANA BREAD

Ingredients:

1 tablespoon ground flaxseeds

3 tablespoons warm water

11/2 cups buckwheat flour

11/2 tablespoons baking powder

1 teaspoon cinnamon

1/2 teaspoon nutmeg

1/2 teaspoon ginger

1 teaspoon kosher salt

1 small zucchini grated (about 1 cup)

2 ripe bananas smashed

1/2 cup milk (or whichever milk works best for you)

11/2 tablespoons melted coconut oil (feel free to substitute a different kind of oil)

1 teaspoon vanilla extract

Directions

Heat oven to 350°F. Grease a 5 x 9 loaf pan with a cooking spray or oil of your choice. In a small bowl mix the ground flaxseed with the warm water and let sit for 10 to 5 minutes. This will act as a binding agent for your bread.

In a large bowl add the buckwheat flour, baking powder, spices and salt, and combine well. Squeeze the excess water out of the zucchini by wrapping it in cheese cloth or a tea towel and squeezing. Add the drained zucchini, bananas, milk, coconut oil, vanilla extract, and flax water mix to the dry ingredients. Stir until well combined and then pour into the loaf pan. Bake for 60 minutes.

DR. LANG'S HEALING SOUP

2 tablespoons miso paste

1 quart water, filtered

2 cups organic broccoli, chopped

2 cups organic carrots, chopped

1 tablespoon organic ginger, minced 4–6 cloves organic garlic, minced 1/8–1/4 cup tamari, to taste

1–2 tablespoons

Sesame oil

1 cup quinoa

Optional:

Onions, minced

Turmeric

Cilantro, minced

Directions

Heat water and add miso paste. Simmer, but do not allow water to boil. Allow paste to dissolve. When dissolved, add broccoli, carrots, ginger, garlic, tamari, sesame oil, and quinoa. Cook until vegetables are tender (30 to 60 minutes).

For easy digestion and optimal absorption, blend the soup. This will break down the broccoli and carrots even further for ease of digestion. Taste and add tamari or sesame oil as desired for flavor.

The ingredients in this dish contain numerous benefits to a balanced gut. Elements like miso paste and tamari include helpful enzymes, while broccoli, carrots, and garlic contain important nutrients and boost liver health.

CURRY TURMERIC LEEK SOUP

Ingredients:

3 tablespoons olive oil

2 leeks, sliced

5 cloves elephant garlic, sliced into large slices 1/2 head Napa cabbage

1 bok choy, chopped

1 quart chicken broth

1 can diced tomatoes

3 teaspoons curry powder or more to taste

1 teaspoon turmeric powder

1 teaspoon fish sauce

1/2 teaspoon organic lemon juice

Sea salt, to taste

Directions

Add olive oil to large saucepan or soup pot on medium low heat. Add leeks and elephant garlic and sauté until medium soft. Increase heat to medium and add cabbage and bok choy and sauté for 3 to 5 minutes. Then add all other ingredients, cover, and simmer on medium to low heat until flavors mingle and vegetables are cooked but still maintain their crunch.

BUTTERNUT SQUASH SOUP

Ingredients:

2 medium butternut squash, peeled, halved, seeded, and cubed 1 cup sweet onion, chopped

1 teaspoon fresh ginger, grated

Approximately 1/4 cup maple syrup

1/4 teaspoon ground nutmeg

1/4 teaspoon ground cinnamon

1⁄4 teaspoon ground cardamom

41⁄2 cups homemade chicken stock

Coarse salt and freshly ground pepper, to taste

1⁄4 cup heavy cream (optional)

1 tablespoon new fresh chives or parsley (optional)

Directions

Steam the squash. Fry onion and ginger and add the spices and chicken stock when the onions are translucent. Blend everything in a blender and serve hot, garnished with either chives or parsley. The soup may be stored and refrigerated for up to three days, or frozen for long as two months.

GRANDMA'S CHICKEN SOUP

Ingredients:

1⁄2 organic chicken

Cinnamon stick (about 6 inches length)

1 dried bay leaf

1 lemon (optional)

Salt, to taste (approximately 2 teaspoons)

Directions

Place the half chicken in a medium pot and add enough water to cover it by 1/2 an inch. Turn the heat on medium-high and bring it to a boil. As it is coming to a boil, take a ladle to skim impurities and fat that rise to the top. Do this until the water appears clear. Add the bay leaf, cinnamon and salt, cover. Reduce to a simmer and cook for 75 minutes. Once it is done, remove the chicken and the cinnamon stick. Taste to see if you need to add more salt and enjoy your delicious, organic clear broth.

For added variety, try some variations on the broth. Add a handful of washed, rinse rice to the broth and simmer for an additional 15 minutes. Once done, take a hand blender and blend it all together. Add diced carrots and half a diced yam to the broth and simmer for an additional 20 minutes, until soft, and add shredded chicken.

Tip: I like to squeeze half a lemon into my bowl but only do that if you can handle the acidity.

I lived off this soup while hospitalized, and for 3 months afterwards once I got home. I loved this soup because it grew with me and became more complex as my diet expanded. I initially just had the broth for a week (my family ate a lot of chicken that week). Then, my grandma would add rice to it and blend it to thicken up the soup for me. Once I gained more strength, I was able to add some shredded pieces of chicken and some carrots and sweet potato pieces. This is one of the soups I still revert to when I have had a bad food reaction or a flare up. I hope this soothes your insides, as it has mine.

LENTIL APRICOT SOUP

Ingredients:

3 tablespoons olive oil

1 onion, chopped

2 cloves garlic, minced

1/3 cup dried apricots, minced 11/2 cups red lentils

5 cups vegetable broth or chicken broth

1/2 teaspoon ground cumin

1/2 teaspoon dried thyme

3 plum tomatoes, peeled, seeded and chopped 2 tablespoons fresh lemon juice

Salt, to taste

Ground black pepper, to taste

Directions:

Sauté onion, garlic, and apricots in olive oil. Add lentils and stock. Bring to a boil, then add spices, reduce heat, and simmer for 30 minutes, covered and stirring occasionally. Add tomatoes and simmer 10 minutes more. Add lemon juice and puree half of the soup in the blender. Add pureed half back into the remaining soup and serve warm.

LENTIL SOUP

Makes 12 cups

Ingredients:

1 pound brown lentils

Water

1/4 pound salt pork

1/2 cup onion, chopped

1 cup celery and leaves, chopped 1/2 cup carrots, chopped

1 clove garlic, chopped

1 bay leaf, crumbled

1 teaspoon honey

1/4 teaspoon thyme leaves

2 tablespoons butter

2 tablespoons flour

1 tablespoon lemon juice Scallions, thinly sliced

Wash lentils. Soak overnight in enough water to cover the lentils. Drain soaking water and measure. Add additional water to make 21⁄2 quarts. Combine lentils, measured water, and salt pork in soup pot. Bring to a boil. Reduce heat and simmer for 2 1⁄2 hours. Add chopped vegetables, garlic, bay leaf, honey, and thyme. Simmer for another 1 to 1 1⁄2 hours.

Remove salt pork from soup pot and put in blender jar with a cup of soup liquid. Blend until smooth. Return to soup pot. In another pan, add butter and blend in flour. Add 2 cups of hot soup to flour mixture and bring to a boil, stirring constantly. Return to soup and stir in lemon

juice. Heat to serving temperature and season to taste with salt. Serve garnished with sliced scallions.

YUMMY KALE SOUP

Prep Time: 40 minutes Serves 4

Ingredients:

1 medium onion, chopped

4 cloves garlic, chopped

5 cups chicken or vegetable broth

1 medium carrot, diced into 1⁄4-inch cubes (about 1 cup) 1 cup diced celery

2 red potatoes, diced into 1⁄2-inch cubes

3 cups kale, rinsed, stems removed and chopped very fine 2 teaspoons dried thyme

2 teaspoons dried sage

Salt and pepper, to taste

Directions

Chop garlic and onions and let sit for 5 minutes to bring out their hidden health benefits.

Heat 1 tablespoon of broth in a medium soup pot. Sauté onion in broth over medium heat for about 5 minutes, stirring frequently. Add garlic and continue to sauté for another minute. Add broth, carrots, and celery and bring to a boil on high heat.

Once it comes to a boil, reduce heat to a simmer and continue to cook for another 5 minutes. Add potatoes and cook until tender, about 15 more minutes. Add kale and rest of ingredients and cook another 5 minutes. If you want to simmer for a longer time for extra flavor and richness, you may need to add a little more broth.

TIP: OIL PULLING

Contributed by Sarah

I first heard about oil pulling from a friend, and when my new GI told me that she does it every morning for 20 minutes, I was already sold. Now I do it every day and have noticed a huge difference in my teeth and gums.

What is oil pulling, you ask? It began in India thousands of years ago as an Ayurvedic remedy using natural substances to detoxify teeth and gums, supporting better oral health. Oil pulling also aids with reducing any inflammation in the mouth.

Some of the other benefits of oil pulling: • Prevents bad breath

• Increases energy

• Clears mind

• Decreases headaches • Clears sinuses

• Alleviates allergies

• Promotes better sleep • Clears skin

• Regulates menstrual cycles • Improves lymphatic system • Improves PMS symptoms

Want to join in on the fun? Here's how you do it: Take 1 tablespoon of organic coconut pressed oil (or sesame oil) and place it in your mouth. Swish it around for 20 minutes (no more). The lipids in the oil mix with your saliva and begin to pull toxins out of your mouth. Make sure not to swallow the oil! It will be full of toxins. Once the 20 minutes is up, spit it out and brush your teeth, rinsing your mouth thoroughly. I reserve a separate toothbrush for this. Your goal is to spit out all those harmful bacteria, fungus, and other organisms out of your mouth. Do this daily!

FRESH MINESTRONE SOUP

Serves 4

Ingredients:

1 onion, chopped

1 garlic clove, crushed

Pinch oregano

1 teaspoon margarine, melted

1 small potato, peeled and diced 1 carrot, diced

1/4 pound green beans, diced

1 stalk celery

1 small tomato

Some parsley, chopped

1 small leek (optional)

1/2 can mushrooms (optional)

1/2 cup corn (optional)

2 okras, cut (optional)

1/2 cup zucchini, sliced (optional)

1/4 cup cabbage, shredded (optional)

Directions

Combine onion, garlic, and oregano with margarine. Cook over low heat until onion is golden. Add 2 cups water and bring to a boil. Add vegetables with the firmest added first. Simmer on low heat until vegetables are tender, but still crisp. Serve in warm soup bowls, thickly garnished with parsley.

COLD CUCUMBER SOUP

Serves 6–8

Ingredients:

3 large cucumbers

1/2 onion, sliced thin

2 tablespoons butter, unsalted

1/2 cup bay leaves

1 tablespoon white rice flour

3 cups low-sodium, fat-free chicken broth 1 teaspoon kosher salt

1 cup almond milk, unsweetened

2 tablespoons lemon juice, fresh or bottled 1/2 teaspoon dill weed, fresh or dried

11/2–2 cups dairy-free sour cream Additional dill (for garnish)

Directions

Peel two of the cucumbers. Slice and sauté cucumbers in butter along with the onions and bay leaves until tender, but not brown. Blend in the flour. Add broth stirring until smooth. Add salt and simmer covered for 25 minutes. Discard bay leaves.

Puree in food processor or blender. Pour through a strainer and discard any solids. Chill well. (The soup can be frozen at this point, or refrigerated for up to 2 days.) The day of serving; skim off any fat on the surface. Add almond milk, lemon juice, and dill weed to the chilled mixture. Peel the remaining cucumber; cut it in half length wise, scoop out the seeds, and coarsely grate. Cover and refrigerate until serving time. This can be done 1–2 hours ahead.

Place about 1 heaping tablespoon of grated cucumber in the bottom of each bowl. Add soup and a dollop of sour cream.

FARMERS' MARKET SOUP

Serves 6

Ingredients:

Stock

1 medium carrot, minced 1 stalk celery, minced

2 medium onions, minced 1 medium shallot, minced 1 medium leek, minced

3 cloves garlic, crushed and unpeeled

7 cups homemade chicken broth (or use low-sodium canned broth) 6 peppercorns

1 sprig fresh thyme

5 parsley stems

Nonstick spray

Soup

2 medium leeks, white and light green parts only, halved lengthwise and cut into 1-inch lengths

6 small red potatoes, scrubbed, cut into 3/4-inch chunks

1 cup frozen peas, thawed

2 cups packed baby spinach

2 tablespoons chopped fresh parsley leaves 1 tablespoon chopped fresh tarragon leaves Salt and fresh ground black pepper, to taste

Directions

Stock

Completely wash and clean all vegetables used in stock (and soup). Combine the carrot, celery, onions, shallot, leek, and garlic in a heavy- bottomed stock pot. Lightly spray the vegetables with cooking spray, toss, and coat. Cover and cook the vegetables over medium heat, stirring until slightly softened and translucent, about 6 minutes. Add the broth, peppercorns, thyme, and parsley stems. Increase the heat to medium high and bring to a simmer. Continue until stock is flavorful (about 15 minutes). Strain the stock, discarding solids.

Soup

Bring the stock to a simmer in a large heavy pot over medium heat. Add the prepared leeks and potatoes and simmer until potatoes are tender, about 9 minutes. Stir in peas, spinach, parsley, and tarragon. Season to taste with salt and pepper.

EXCELLENT SAVORY TOFU STEW

Serves 6–8

Ingredients:

1/4 cup olive or vegetable oil

3 onions, thinly sliced

4 carrots, thinly sliced

4–5 stalks celery, thinly sliced

2–3 cloves garlic, minced or pressed

1 cup firm tofu (press out excess water)

1 1/2 cups zucchini or yellow squash, 1/4-inch slices 2 fresh tomatoes, diced

1 tablespoon dried basil

2 bay leaves

2 cups tomato juice

1/3 cup soy sauce (or tamari)

Directions

Heat oil in a large lidded pot over medium heat. Add onion, carrots, celery, and garlic, cooking until onions are transparent. Add tofu, zucchini or squash, and tomatoes. Simmer a bit, and then add herbs. Simmer for 2–3 minutes. Pour in tomato juice and soy sauce; stir. Reduce heat to low, cover pot, and simmer for one hour.

JULIE'S PISTOU

Serves 4

Ingredients:

1 tablespoon butter

1 medium onion, diced

1 leek, diced

2 large tomatoes, peeled, seeded, and crushed

4 cups chicken or vegetarian stock or water

1/2 pound fresh green beans

3 potatoes, cut into bite-sized pieces

Approximately 1/4 pound of spaghetti, broken in half 2 cloves garlic, crushed

Several basil leaves, crushed

2 tablespoons olive oil

2–3 tablespoons broth (chicken or vegetarian)

4 tablespoons Parmesan cheese, grated Salt and pepper, to taste

Directions

In a medium heavy pot over medium-low heat, melt butter and slowly cook onion and leek. Add tomatoes. Add stock or water to pot and bring to a boil. Add fresh green beans and potatoes. Season with salt and pepper, to taste. When vegetables are almost cooked (about 15 minutes) add spaghetti. Reduce heat and finish cooking very slowly.

While cooking, to make the pesto, pound the garlic with several basil leaves. Add, while still pounding, olive oil and 2–3 tablespoons chicken or vegetarian broth. Serve soup, dividing pesto and Parmesan cheese between portions.

White beans, zucchini, and carrots can all be added; if you are in a hurry, cheat and use already prepared basil pesto.

Another childhood favorite, this was always a late summer or early harvest meal based on what was in the garden.

Salads and Side Dises

ARUGULA, AVOCADO AND CUCUMBER SALAD

Serves 3–4 people

Ingredients:

Dressing

1/2 teaspoon salt

2 tablespoons balsamic vinegar

3 tablespoons extra virgin olive oil 1/4 teaspoon garlic powder

Salad

2 large handfuls of organic baby arugula

3 organic, Persian cucumbers, peeled and diced 1 ripe organic avocado, diced.

Directions

Place all the dressing ingredients in a jar and shake. Clean the vegetables then place the vegetables in a medium bowl and toss with as much dressing as you would like.

KALE AND CARROT SALAD

Ingredients:

Salad

1 bunch kale, chopped

5 large carrots, sliced

2 tablespoons sesame seeds 2 tablespoons hemp seeds Sea salt, to taste

Dressing

1 tablespoon sesame oil

1 tablespoon olive oil

1/3 cup brown rice vinegar

1 teaspoon pure maple syrup

Directions

Steam carrots and kale until soft, but still crunchy and let cool. Mix with seeds, coat with dressing mixture, and store in the refrigerator. Flavors will mix if left overnight. Serve chilled.

Tip: If seeds like sesame or hemp cause digestive problems, omit them from the recipe or do not make this recipe. I also recommend grinding the seeds first (a coffee grinder works well).

EASY SALMON SALAD

Ingredients:

2 cans wild boneless, skinless salmon

1/2 cup mayonnaise, organic

1/2 cup minced carrots

1/2 cup minced apples

1/4 cup sweet relish, organic and sweetened naturally

Mix all ingredients in a large bowl. Serve chilled with crackers, as a salad, or alone.

SPINACH SALAD

Serves 4

Ingredients:

Dressing

2 tablespoons olive oil

1 tablespoon cider vinegar

1 tablespoon chopped fresh parsley 1 teaspoon lemon juice

1/4 teaspoon maple syrup

Salad

1 cup cooked rice noodles

2 cups torn raw spinach or salad mix

3/4 cup sliced celery

1/4 cup sliced green onions

1 medium tomato or 1 cup cherry tomatoes

1/2 cup raw snow peas

1 cup seedless grapes (optional)

1/2 pound cooked shrimp or 8-ounce chicken breast (optional)

Place all dressing ingredients in pint jar, close with lid, and shake well. Cook noodles according to package directions, but do not add salt to water. Drain, rinse, and cool. Place torn fresh spinach in large salad bowl. Chop celery and green onions. Slice fresh tomato into small wedges or cut cherry tomatoes into halves. Wash grapes (if using) and snow peas and add all to salad bowl.

If using cooked fresh or frozen shrimp, remove peels and veins. If using cooked chicken, cut into bite-size pieces using separate cutting board. Add to salad bowl. Place drained and cooled pasta in salad bowl. Shake dressing and pour over salad. Toss with salad tongs or two large spoons.

CHICKPEA SALAD WITH LEMON AND PARMESAN

Serves 2

Ingredients:

69

1 (15-ounce) can chickpeas, drained and rinsed

1 teaspoon fresh lemon juice

11⁄2 teaspoon olive oil

1⁄4 cup loosely packed shredded Parmigianino Reggiano, or dairy- free substitute

1–2 finely minced garlic cloves (optional) Pinch of salt

Directions

Combine all ingredients in a bowl, and stir gently to mix. Taste, and adjust seasoning as necessary. Serve immediately, or chill, covered, until serving.

This little salad only has five ingredients, so make sure that they're all of good quality. There's no room for second-rate pantry closet cast-offs here, so don't even think about it! First of all, be sure to use a good brand of chickpeas. Also, get out your best olive oil—one you'd want to eat from a spoon, if you're into that sort of thing. This salad keeps well in the fridge and is, in my humble opinion, best eaten cold.

WARM SALMON SALAD AND CRISPY POTATOES

Serves 4

Ingredients:

2 tablespoons extra virgin olive oil, divided

2 small yellow-fleshed potatoes, scrubbed and cut into 1/8-inch slices 1/2 teaspoon salt, divided

1 medium shallot, thinly sliced

2 teaspoons rice vinegar

1/4 cup buttermilk

2 (7-ounce) cans boneless, skinless salmon, drained

4 cups arugula

Directions

Heat 1 tablespoon of olive oil in a large nonstick skillet over medium- high heat. Add potatoes and cook, turning once, until brown and crispy (5–6 minutes per side). Transfer to a plate and season with 1/4 teaspoon salt; cover with foil to keep warm. Combine the remaining 1 tablespoon oil, 1/4 teaspoon salt, shallot, and vinegar in a small saucepan. Bring to a boil over medium heat. Remove from heat and whisk in buttermilk. Place salmon in a medium bowl and toss with the warm dressing. Divide arugula among four plates and top with the potatoes and salmon.

HIPPY YUM-YUM SALAD
Serves 4

Ingredients:

1 red onion

1/3 cup chives

1 medium-sized red potato 1/2 large sweet potato

1/3 cup olive oil

Pinch of fresh rosemary

2 medium heads of romaine lettuce 2 shredded, sliced or peeled carrots 1 avocado

1/2 cup hummus (see this page)

1/3 cup balsamic vinegar Pinch of fresh dill

Juice of half a lemon

Directions

Cut up onion, chives, and the two potatoes (very thinly sliced). Dump olive oil in a large frying pan. Put in onion, potato, chives, and rosemary into frying pan. Stir occasionally.

Cut up romaine lettuce, carrots, and avocado into a bowl. When frying pan ingredients have browned and are sizzling, dump them in with the salad. Pour in balsamic vinegar and mix with hummus and lemon juice, and sprinkle with dill.

Salmon, sardines, chicken, or chickpeas can be added for protein.

CARROT, APPLE, AND RAISIN SALAD*

Serves 8

Ingredients:

1 large (8-ounce) apple, peeled and cored

2 teaspoons lemon juice

3/4 pound raw carrots

3 tablespoons dark raisins

1/3 cup dairy-free sour cream

3 tablespoons almond or coconut milk 1 teaspoon maple syrup

1/4 teaspoon ground cinnamon

1/4 teaspoon ground nutmeg

Directions

Peel, core, and shred apple. Place apple in large mixing bowl and toss with lemon juice. Peel and grate carrots. Toss carrots and raisins with apple. Mix non-fat sour cream with milk, sweetener, cinnamon, and nutmeg in small bowl. Pour over carrot mixture, toss with rubber scraper to coat; divide into serving bowls. Cover tightly with plastic wrap and chill for 1 hour or more.

For preparing in food processor:

Fit food processor with metal chopping blade. Place non-fat sour cream, milk, lemon juice, sweetener, cinnamon, and nutmeg in bowl of food processor. Blend on and off to mix. Unplug food processor and remove metal chopping blade, leaving sour cream mixture in bottom of mixing bowl. Fit food processor with grating tool. Grate carrots and apples directly into sour cream mixture. Turn off food processor and remove grating tool. Turn mixture into serving bowl. Sprinkle raisins over top of mixture and toss to blend.

Cover tightly with plastic wrap. Chill 1 hour or more before serving.

CRISPY BAKED BRUSSELS WITH CARROTS
Serves 4

Ingredients:

1 pound whole Brussels sprouts (approximately 1 16-ounce bag), cut into quarters

2 cups (about 4–5 medium sized) carrots, peeled and sliced fairly thin

1/3 cup extra virgin olive oil 3/4 teaspoon salt

74

1/2 teaspoon garlic powder 1/4 teaspoon pepper

Juice of half a lemon

Directions

Preheat oven to 400°F. Mix all of all of the ingredients except the lemon in a bowl. Place the mixed ingredients onto a foiled baking (cookie) sheet and spread out evenly. Bake for 20 minutes, then take a look and toss around the Brussels sprouts and carrots, turning them over if browning has begun on the bottom. Rotate the baking sheet; some ovens have more heat in the back then in the front and we want to distribute the heat evenly. Cook for an additional 10 minutes. Remove the baking sheet and squeeze on the juice of half a lemon on top of the Brussels sprouts and carrots. Lightly toss and serve.

ALMOND CHEESE SPREAD

Ingredients:

11/2 cups almond meal

1/4 fresh lemon juice

1/4 cup extra virgin olive oil 1 garlic clove minced

1/4 teaspoon of thyme

1/2 cup water

Add all of the ingredients to a food processor and blend for 5 minutes. Line a strainer with a couple of layers of cheesecloth, pour the mixture into the cheesecloth and collect the ends of the cloth and tie together, making a little sack. Leave the cheese in the strainer, place the strainer on a plate and refrigerate overnight.

The next day, preheat the oven to 350°F. Generously spray a small oven safe bowl with nonstick spray. Gently remove the cheese from the cheesecloth and place in the bowl. Bake the almond spread for 40 minutes until lightly brown on the top. Remove it from the oven and let it cool.

Serve with your favorite gluten-free crackers or spread on a brown rice tortilla. This dish will last about a week in the fridge.

This is another of my mom's recipes. I am blessed to have a creative mom, and because I miss cheese at times, she decided to create a "cheese" I can eat. This one is a bit more time consuming, but makes for a fun activity to do on a weekend.